My Air Fryer Recipe Book

Easy & Healthy Recipes to Make Unforgettable First Courses

Kira Hamm

TABLE OF CONTENT

Mustard Marina Ted Beef

Preparation Time: 10 Minutes

Cooking Time: 45 Minutes

Servings: 6

Ingredients:

- 3 lb. beef roast
- 6 bacon strips
- 1-3/4 beef stock
- 2 tbsp. butter
- 3/4 cup red wine
- 1 tbsp. horseradish
- 3 cloves garlic (minced)
- 1 tbsp. mustard
- Salt and pepper, to taste

Directions:

1. Preheat the air fryer to 4000F.
2. In a bowl, add the butter, horseradish, mustard, garlic, salt, garlic, and mix. Rub the beef with the mixture.
3. Arrange the bacon on a cutting board, add the meat on top and wrap the beef with the bacon strips. Put it into the air fryer then

cook for 15 minutes. Remove the beef roast and transfer to a pan.

4. Add the stock and wine to the pan, lower the temperature to 3600F and cook for 30minutes.

5. Carve the beef and serve.

Nutrition : Calories: 350kcal, Fat: 9g, Carb: 27g, Proteins: 29g

Chinese Steak and Broccoli

Preparation Time: 30 Minutes

Cooking Time: 12 Minutes

Servings: 8

Ingredients:

- 3/4 lb. steak cut into strips
- 1/3 cup oyster sauce
- 1/3 cup sherry
- 1 lb. broccoli florets
- 1 tsp. soy sauce
- 2 tsp. sesame oil
- 1 tsp. sugar
- 1 garlic clove (minced)
- 1 tbsp. olive oil

Directions:

1. Preheat the air fryer to 3800F.
2. In a bowl, mix the oyster sauce, sesame oil, sherry, soy sauce, and sugar. Add the beef and mix; leave to marinate for 30 minutes.
3. Transfer the meat to a pan that fits into the air fryer, add the broccoli, garlic, oil, and toss together. Cook for 12 minutes.
4. Uncover the air fryer, serve, and enjoy.

Nutrition: Calories: 330kcal, Fat: 12g, Carb: 17g, Proteins: 23g

Beef Brisket and Onion Sauce

Preparation Time: 10 Minutes

Cooking Time: 2 Hours

Servings: 6

Ingredients:

- 4 lb. beef brisket
- 1 lb. yellow onion (chopped)
- 1/2 lb. chopped celery
- 1 lb. chopped carrot
- 4 cups of water
- 8 earl gray tea bags
- Salt and black pepper to taste
- 4 lb. beef brisket
- 1 lb. yellow onion (chopped)
- 1/2 lb. chopped celery
- 1 lb. chopped carrot
- 4 cups of water
- 8 earl gray tea bags
- Salt and black pepper to taste

Directions:

1. Preheat the air fryer to 3000F.

2. Put water in a pan that fits into the air fryer. Add the onions, celery, carrots, salt, and pepper. Stir and allow to simmer over medium-high heat.
3. Add the beef brisket, 8 earl grey tea bags, and stir. Put it into the air fryer then cook for 1 hour 30 minutes.
4. Meanwhile, place a pan over medium-high heat, add vegetable oil, and heat until shimmering. Add the sweet onion and sauté for 10 minutes. Add the remaining sauce ingredients and cook for 10 minutes. Remove and discard the teabags.
5. Cut and serve the beef brisket with the onion sauce.

Nutrition: Calories: 400kcal, Fat: 12g, Carb: 26g, Proteins: 34g

Beef Curry

Preparation Time: 6 Minutes

Cooking Time: 44 Minutes

Servings: 4

Ingredients:

- 2 lb. beef (cut into cubes)
- 2 tbsp. tomato sauce
- 3 medium potatoes (cut into cubes)
- 2 yellow onions chopped
- 2 tbsp. olive oil
- 1 tbsp. wine mustard
- 2 garlic cloves (minced)
- 2-1/2 tbsp. curry
- 10 oz. can coconut milk
- Salt and black pepper to taste

Directions:

1. Preheat the air fryer to 3600F.
2. Place a pan over medium heat (make sure the pan fits into your air fryer), add oil, and heat until shimmering. Add the onions and garlic, cook for 4 minutes or until translucent. Add the beef, curry powder,

tomato sauce, coconut milk, salt, and pepper.

3. Stir and transfer to the air fryer; set the Time for 40 minutes.

4. Serve and enjoy.

Nutrition: Calories: 231kcal, Fat: 15g, Carb: 20g, Proteins: 27g

Garlic and Bell Pepper Beef

Preparation Time:30 Minutes

Cooking Time: 21 Minutes

Servings: 4

Ingredients:

- 11 oz. steak fillets (sliced)
- 1/2 cup beef stock
- 2 tbsp. olive oil
- 2 tbsp. fish sauce
- 4 cloves garlic (pressed)
- 1 red pepper (cut into thin strips)
- 4 green onions (sliced)
- 1 tbsp. sugar
- 2 tsp. corn flour
- Black pepper to taste

Directions:

1. In a pan, add beef, oil, garlic, black pepper, and bell pepper, stir, cover, and keep in the refrigerator for 30 minutes.
2. Preheat the air fryer to 3600F.
3. Put the pan to the air fryer and cook for 14 minutes. In a bowl, mix sugar and fish

sauce, pour over the beef and cook for an additional 7 minutes.

4. Serve and enjoy.

Nutrition: Calories: 243kcal, Fat: 3g, Carb: 24g, Proteins: 38g

Beef and Green Onion Marinade

Preparation Time:10 Minutes

Cooking Time: 20 Minutes

Servings: 4

Ingredients:

- 1 lb. lean beef
- 1 cup of soy sauce
- 5 garlic cloves (minced)
- 1/4 cup sesame seeds
- 1/2 cup of water
- 1 tsp. black pepper
- 1/4 cup brown sugar
- 1 cup green onion

Directions:

1. In a bowl, add soy sauce, onions, sugar, water, garlic, sesame seed, and pepper, whisk. Add the beef and toss to coat, leave for 10 minutes.
2. Preheat the air fryer to 3900F, drain the beef, and transfer to the air fryer. Cook for 20 minutes.
3. Serve with salad and enjoy.

Nutrition : Calories: 329kcal, Fat: 8g, Carb: 24g, Proteins: 22g

Beef Roasted Wine Sauce

Preparation Time: 10 Minutes

Cooking Time: 45 Minutes

Servings: 6

Ingredients:

- 3 lb. beef roast
- carrot (chopped)
- 3 oz. red wine
- 1/2 tsp. smoked paprika
- 5 potatoes chopped
- 1/2 tsp. salt
- 1 yellow onion (chopped)
- 4 garlic cloves (pressed)
- 17 oz. beef stock
- 1/2 tsp. chicken salt

Directions:

1. Preheat the air fryer to 3600F.
2. In a bowl, add salt, paprika, and chicken salt, stir. Rub the beef with the mixture and transfer to a plan that will fit into the air dryer.
3. Add the remaining ingredients and cook for 45 minutes.

4. Enjoy and serve.

Nutrition: Calories: 304kcal, Fat: 20g, Carb: 18g, Proteins: 32g

Short Ribs and Beer Sauce

Preparation Time:15 Minutes

Cooking Time: 43 Minutes

Servings: 6

Ingredients:

- 4 lb. short ribs (cut into small pieces)
- 1 dried Portobello mushroom
- 1 yellow onion (chopped)
- 1 cup chicken stock
- 6 thyme sprigs (chopped)
- 1/4 cup tomato paste
- 1 bay leaf
- 1 cup dark beer
- Salt and pepper to taste

Directions:

1. Preheat the air fryer to 3500F.
2. In a pan that fits into your air fryer, heat oil over medium heat, add onion, stock, tomato paste, beer, mushroom, bay leaf, and thyme. Simmer for 3-5minutes.
3. Add the rib and transfer to the air fryer, cook for 40 minutes.
4. Bon appetite!

Nutrition: Calories: 300kcal, Fat: 7g, Carb: 18g, Proteins: 23g

Beef and Cabbage Mix

Preparation Time:10 Minutes

Cooking Time: 40 Minutes

Servings: 6

Ingredients:

- 2-1/2 lb. beef brisket
- 3 garlic cloves, preferably pressed
- 1 cup beef stock
- 1 cabbage cut into wedges
- 2 bay leaves
- 4 carrots, chopped
- 2 turnips (cut into smaller pieces)
- Salt and black pepper to taste

Directions:

1. Preheat the air fryer to 3600F.
2. Put the beef in a pan, add the stock, salt, pepper, carrots, cabbage, bay leaves, garlic, turnip, stir, transfer to the air fryer, and cover. Cook for 40 minutes.
3. Serve and enjoy.

Nutrition: Calories: 355kcal, Fat: 16g, Carb: 18g, Proteins: 24g

Short Ribs and Special Sauce

Preparation Time:10 Minutes

Cooking Time: 46 Minutes

Servings: 4

Ingredients:

- 4 lb. short ribs
- 1/2 cup of soy sauce
- 3 cloves garlic (pressed)
- 1/2 cup of water
- 2 tbsp. sesame oil
- 1/4 cup of rice wine
- 3 ginger slices
- 1/4 cup pear juice
- 1 tsp. vegetable oil
- 2 green onions chopped

Directions:

1. Preheat the air fryer to 3500F.
2. Heat oil in a pan, then put green onions, garlic, and ginger, stir and cook for 1 minute.

3. Add the rib and the remaining ingredients, transfer to the air fryer and cook for 35 minutes.
4. Serve and enjoy.

Nutrition: Calories: 321kcal, Fat: 12g, Carb: 20g, Proteins: 14g

Beef Patty in Mushroom Sauce

Preparation Time:15 Minutes

Cooking Time: 22 Minutes

Servings: 6

Ingredients:

- 2 lb. ground beef
- 3/4 cup flour
- 1 tbsp. onion flakes
- 1/2 tsp. garlic powder
- 1/4 cup beef stock
- 1 tbsp. chopped parsley
- 1 tbsp. soy sauce
- Salt and pepper to taste
- 1/2 cup beef stock
- 1/2 tsp. soy sauce
- 2 cups mushroom, sliced
- 2 tbsp. butter
- 1 cup yellow onion, chopped
- 2 tbsp. bacon fat
- 1/4 cup sour cream
- Salt and black pepper to taste

Directions:

1. Preheat the air fryer to 3500F.

2. In a bowl, mix beef, pepper, salt, garlic powder, 1 tbsp soy sauce, ¼ cup beef stock, parsley, onions flakes, and flour. Stir and shape six patties. Move it into the air fryer and cook for 14 minutes.

3. While the patties are still cooking, heat butter in a pan on medium heat, add the mushroom and cook for 4 minutes with constant stirring. Add onions and cook for another 4 minutes, add the soy sauce, sour cream, and simmer. Remove from heat.

4. Serve patties with mushroom sauce.

Nutrition: Calories: 235kcal, Fat: 23g, Carb: 6g, Proteins: 32g

Greek Beef Meatballs Salad

Preparation Time: 10 Minutes

Cooking Time: 10 Minutes

Servings: 6

Ingredients:

- 17 oz. ground beef
- 1 cup baby spinach
- 5 bread slices, cubed
- 1/4 cup parsley
- 1/4 cup milk
- 1/4 cup chopped mint
- 1 yellow onion (minced)
- 1 tbsp. olive oil
- 7 oz. cherry tomatoes (halved)
- 1 egg whisked
- 2 garlic cloves (minced)
- 2-1/2 tsp. dried oregano
- Cooking spray
- Salt and pepper to taste

Directions:

1. Preheat the air fryer to 3700F.

2. Add the bread and milk and allow to soak for 3 minutes. Squeeze and transfer to another bowl.
3. To the bread in the bowl, add egg, salt, pepper, mint, parsley, garlic, and onion. Stir and shaped into balls using ice-cream scooper.
4. Spray the meatballs with cooking spray, place in your air fryer and cook for 10 minutes.
5. In a bowl, mix spinach, cucumber, and tomatoes. Add the meatball, oil, pepper, salt, lemon juice, and yogurt. Toss, and serve.

Nutrition : Calories: 200kcal, Fat: 4g, Carb: 13g, Proteins: 27g

Beef Stuffed Squash

Preparation Time: 10 Minutes

Cooking Time: 40 Minutes

Servings: 2

Ingredients:

- 1 lb. ground beef
- 1 tsp. dried oregano
- 1 spaghetti squash (pricked)
- 3 garlic cloves (minced)
- 28 oz. canned tomatoes (chopped)
- 1 Portobello mushroom (sliced)
- 1/2 tsp. dried thyme
- 1 green bell pepper (chopped)
- 1/4 tsp. cayenne pepper
- 1 yellow onion (diced)
- Salt and pepper to taste

Directions:

1. Preheat the air fryer to 3500F, transfer the spaghetti squash into the air fryer, and cook for 20 minutes. Remove and transfer to the cutting board and cut into halves. Remove and discard the seeds.

2. Heat a pan over medium heat, add the beef, garlic, onions, mushroom, stir and cook until the meat is golden brown. Add the remaining ingredients except for the squash and allow them to cook for 10 minutes.

3. Stuff the squash with the beef mix and transfer into the air fryer; cook for 10 minutes at 3600F.

4. Serve and enjoy.

Nutrition: Calories: 260kcal, Fat: 7g, Carb: 14g, Proteins: 10g

Beef Casserole

Preparation Time:15 Minutes

Cooking Time: 35 Minutes

Servings: 12

Ingredients:

- 2 lb. beef
- 2 tsp. mustard
- 2 cups of grated mozzarella
- 1 tbsp. olive oil
- 2 cups. chopped eggplant
- 28 oz. canned tomatoes (chopped)
- 1 tsp. dried oregano
- 2 tsp. Worcestershire sauce
- 2 tbsp. chopped parsley
- 16 oz. tomato sauce
- Salt and pepper to taste

Directions:

1. Preheat the air fryer to 3600F.
2. In a bowl, add eggplant, salt, pepper, and oil, mix to coat.
3. In a separate bowl, add beef, mustard, salt, pepper, and Worcestershire sauce, stir well. Pour the mixture into a pan that fits into

your air fryer and spread evenly; add the eggplant mix and tomato sauce. Sprinkle with parsley and oregano.

4. Transfer to the air fryer and cook 35 minutes.
5. Serve and enjoy.

Nutrition: Calories: 200kcal, Fat: 12g, Carb: 16g, Proteins: 15g

Burgundy Beef Mix

Preparation Time:10 Minutes

Cooking Time: 1 Hour 5 Minutes

Servings: 7

Ingredients:

- 2 lb. beef chuck roast, cut into smaller cubes
- 4 carrots (chopped)
- 1 cup of water
- 1 cup. beef stock
- 3 tbsp. almond flour
- 2 yellow onions (chopped)
- 1 tbsp. chopped thyme
- 2 celery ribs (chopped)
- 1/2 lb. mushroom (sliced)
- 15 oz. canned tomatoes(chopped)
- 1/2 tsp. mustard powder
- Salt and black pepper to taste

Directions:

1. Preheat the air fryer to 3000F.
2. Place a pot over high heat then place the meat and brown on all sides for 3-5 minutes. Add the tomato, carrot, onions,

celery, mushroom, salt, pepper, mustard, stock, and thyme, stir.

3. In a bowl, add water and flour, stir. Add to the pot and transfer into the air fryer and cook for 1 hour.

4. Serve and enjoy.

Nutrition : Calories: 275kcal, Fat: 13g, Carb: 17g, Proteins: 28g

Sirloin Steaks and Pico de Gallo

Preparation Time:10 Minutes

Cooking Time: 10 Minutes

Servings: 4

Ingredients:

- 4 medium sirloin steak
- 1 tsp. onion powder
- 1/2 tbsp. sweet paprika
- 1 tsp. garlic powder
- 2 tbsp. chili powder
- 1 tsp. ground cumin
- Salt and pepper to taste
- For the Pico de Gallo:
- 2 tomatoes (chopped)
- 2 tbsp. lime juice
- 1 jalapeno (chopped)
- 1 small red onion (chopped)
- 1/4 cup chopped cilantro
- 1 small red onion (diced)
- 1/4 tsp. cumin
- 1 red onion (chopped)

Directions:

1. Preheat the air fryer to 3600F.

2. In a bowl, mix chili powder, onion powder, salt, pepper, garlic powder, paprika, and 1 tsp. cumin. Rub the combination into the both sides of the steak then transfer to your air fryer. Cook for 10 minutes.

3. Mix all the Pico de Gallo ingredients in a bowl and add pepper to taste.

4. Serve the steak with the Pico de Gallo at the side, enjoy.

Nutrition: Calories: 200kcal, Fat: 12g, Carb: 15g, Proteins: 18g

Mexican Beef Mix

Preparation Time: 10 Minutes

Cooking Time: 1 Hour 10 Minutes

Servings: 8

Ingredients:

- 2 lb. beef roast, cubes
- 2 green bell peppers (chopped)
- 6 garlic cloves (minced)
- 2 tbsp. olive oil
- 4 jalapenos (chopped)
- 2 yellow onions (diced)
- 1/2 cup of water
- 1 tsp. dried oregano
- 1 Habanero pepper (chopped)
- 2 tbsp. cilantro (chopped)
- 14 oz. canned tomatoes (chopped)
- 1/2 cup of black olive (pitted and chopped)
- 1 and 1/2 tsp. ground cumin
- Salt and pepper to taste

Directions:

1. Preheat the air fryer to 3000F.

2. In a pan, add all the ingredients and stir, transfer to the air fryer and cook for 1 hour 10 minutes.

3. Serve garnished with olives.

Nutrition: Calories: 305kcal, Fat: 14g, Carb: 1825g, Proteins: g

Coffee Flavored Steak

Preparation Time:10 Minutes

Cooking Time: 15 Minutes

Servings: 4

Ingredients:

- 4 rib-eye steak
- 2 tbsp. garlic powder
- 2 tbsp. chili powder
- 1-1/2 tbsp. ground coffee
- 2 tbsp. onion powder
- 1/2 tbsp. sweet paprika
- Pinch of cayenne pepper
- 1/4 tsp. ground ginger
- Black pepper to taste
- 1/4 tsp. ground coriander

Directions:

1. Preheat the air fryer to 3600F.
2. In a bowl, mix all the fixings excluding the steak and stir. Rub the steak thoroughly with the mixture.
3. Transfer to the air fryer and cook for 15 minutes.
4. Serve and enjoy.

Nutrition: Calories: 160kcal, Fat: 10g, Carb: 14g, Proteins: 12g

Seasoned Beef Roast

Preparation Time: 10 Minutes

Cooking Time: 45 Minutes

Servings: 10

Ingredients:

- 3 pounds beef top roast
- One tablespoon olive oil
- Two tablespoons Montreal steak seasoning

Directions:

1. Coat the roast with oil and then rub with the seasoning generously.
2. With kitchen twines, tie the roast to keep it compact. Arrange the roast onto the cooking tray.
3. Select "Air Fry" and then alter the temperature to 360 degrees F. Set the Timer for 45 minutes and press the "Start."
4. If the display shows "Add Food," insert the cooking tray in the center position.
5. When the display shows "Turn Food," do nothing.

6. When cooking Time is complete, take away the tray from Vortex.
7. Place the roast onto a platter for about 10 minutes before slicing.
8. With a sharp knife, cut the roast into desired sized slices and serve.

Nutrition : Calories 269 Fat 9.9 g Carbs 0 g Fiber 0 g

Simple Beef Sirloin Roast

Preparation Time: 10 Minutes

Cooking Time: 50 Minutes

Servings: 8

Ingredients:

- 2½ pounds sirloin roast
- Salt and ground black pepper, as required

Directions:

1. Rub the roast with salt and black pepper generously.
2. Insert the rotisserie rod through the roast.
3. Insert the rotisserie forks, one on each rod's side, to secure the rod to the chicken.
4. Select "Roast" and then adjust the temperature to 350 degrees F.
5. Set the Timer for 50 minutes and press the "Start."
6. When the display shows "Add Food," press the red lever down.
7. Weight the left side of the rod into the Vortex.

8. Now, turn the rod's left side into the groove along the metal bar so it will not move.

9. Then, close the door and touch "Rotate." Press the red lever to release the rod when cooking Time is complete.

10. Remove from the Vortex.

11. Place the roast onto a platter for about 10 minutes before slicing.

12. With a sharp knife, cut the roast into desired sized slices and serve.

Nutrition : Calories 201 Fat 8.8 g Carbs 0 g Protein 28.9 g

Simple Beef Patties

Preparation Time:10 Minutes

Cooking Time: 13 Minutes

Servings: 4

Ingredients:

- 1 lb. ground beef
- ½ tsp garlic powder
- ¼ tsp onion powder
- Pepper
- Salt

Directions:

1. Preheat the instant vortex air fryer oven to 400 F.
2. Add ground meat, garlic powder, onion powder, pepper, and salt into the mixing bowl and mix until well combined.
3. Make even shape patties from meat mixture and arrange on air fryer pan.
4. Place pan in instant vortex air fryer oven.
5. Cook patties for 10 minutes Turn patties after 5 minutes
6. Serve and enjoy.

Nutrition: Calories 212 Fat 7.1 g Carbs 0.4 g Protein

34.5 g

Easy Beef Roast

Preparation Time:10 Minutes

Cooking Time: 45 Minutes

Servings: 6

Ingredients:

- 2 ½ lbs. beef roast
- 2 tbsp Italian seasoning

Directions:

1. Arrange roast on the rotisserie spite.
2. Rub roast with Italian seasoning, then insert into the instant vortex air fryer oven.
3. Air fry at 350 F for 45 minutes or until the roast's internal temperature reaches 145 F.
4. Slice and serve.

Nutrition: Calories 365 Fat 13.2 g Carbs 0.5 g Protein 57.4 g

Beef Sirloin Roast

Preparation Time: 10 Minutes

Cooking Time: 50 Minutes

Servings: 8

Ingredients:

- 1 tablespoon smoked paprika
- 1 teaspoon ground cumin
- 1 teaspoon garlic powder
- Salt and freshly ground black pepper, to taste
- 2½ pounds sirloin roast

Directions:

1. In a bowl, mix together the spices, salt and black pepper.
2. Rub the roast with spice mixture generously.
3. Place the sirloin roast into the greased baking pan.
4. Press "Power Button" of Power XL Digital Air Fry Oven and turn the dial to select "Air Roast" mode.
5. Press "Time Button" and again turn the dial to set the cooking Time to 50 minutes.

6. Now push "Temp Button" and rotate the dial to set the temperature at 350 degrees F.
7. Press "Start/Pause" button to start.
8. When the unit beeps to show that it is preheated, open the lid and insert baking pan in the oven.
9. When cooking Time is complete, open the lid and place the roast onto a platter for about 10 minutes before slicing.
10. With a sharp knife, cut the beef roast into desired sized slices and serve.

Nutrition: Calories: 260 Fat: 11.9g Sat Fat: 4.4g Carbohydrates: 0.4g Fiber: 0.1g Sugar: 0.1g Protein: 38g

Air Fried Grilled Steak

Preparation Time:6 Minutes

Cooking Time: 40 Minutes

Servings: 2

Ingredients:

- Two sirloin steaks
- 3 tbsp. butter, melted
- 3 tbsp. olive oil
- Salt and pepper, to taste

Directions:

1. Preheat the Smart Air Fryer Oven for 5 minutes at 350°F.
2. Season the sirloin steaks with olive oil, salt, and pepper.
3. Place the beef in the air fryer basket and put the basket into the oven.
4. Select GRILL. Grill for 40 minutes at 350°F.
5. Once cooked, serve with butter.

Nutrition: Calories 1536 Fat 123.7 g Protein 103.4 g

Air Fryer Beef Casserole

Preparation Time: 7 Minutes

Cooking Time: 30 Minutes

Servings: 4

Ingredients:

- One green bell pepper, seeded and chopped
- One onion, chopped
- 1-lb. ground beef
- Three cloves of garlic, minced
- 6 cups eggs, beaten

Directions:

1. Preheat the Smart Air Fryer Oven for 5 minutes at 325°F.
2. In a baking dish, mix the ground beef, onion, garlic, olive oil, and bell pepper.
3. Add beaten eggs to a large bowl.
4. Season the ground beef mixture with salt and pepper and pour in the beaten eggs and give a good stir.
5. Place the dish with the beef and egg mixture in the air fryer.

6. Place the rack on the middle shelf of the Smart Air Fryer Oven.

7. Select BAKE. Set temperature to 325°F, and set Time to 30 minutes.

8. When done, remove from the oven and rest for 5 minutes. Serve warm.

Nutrition: Calories 1520 Fat 125.1 g Protein 87.9 g

Charred Onions & Steak Cube BBQ

Preparation Time:8 Minutes

Cooking Time: 40 Minutes

Servings: 3

Ingredients:

- 1 cup red onions, cut into wedges
- 1 tbsp. dry mustard
- 1 tbsp. olive oil
- 1-lb. boneless beef sirloin, cut into cubes
- Salt and pepper, to taste

Directions:

1. Preheat the air fryer to 390°F.
2. Place the grill rack in the air fryer. Toss all the listed ingredients in a bowl and mix until everything is coated with the seasonings.
3. Place on the grill rack and put the rack in the oven.
4. Select GRILL. Grill for 40 minutes.
5. Halfway through the cooking Time, give a stir to cook evenly.
6. When done, transfer to a plate and enjoy.

Nutrition: Calories 260 Fat 10.7 g Protein 35.5 g

Beef Ribeye Steak

Preparation Time: 6 Minutes

Cooking Time: 10 Minutes

Servings: 4

Ingredients:

- 4 (8-oz.) rib-eye steaks
- 1 tbsp. McCormick Grill Mates Montreal Steak Seasoning
- Salt and pepper, to taste

Directions:

1. Season the steaks with salt, pepper, and seasoning.
2. Place two steaks in the Smart Air Fryer Oven grill rack.
3. Select GRILL and grill for 5 minutes at 400°F.
4. Open the air fryer and flip the steaks. Then cook for an additional 5 minutes.
5. Remove the cooked steaks from the Smart Air Fryer Oven to a plate.
6. Repeat for the remaining two steaks.
7. Serve warm.

Nutrition: Calories 293 Fat 22 g Fiber 0 g Protein 23

Air Fryer Roast Beef

Preparation Time: 7 Minutes

Cooking Time: 20 Minutes

Servings: 6

Ingredients:

- Roast beef
- 1 tbsp. olive oil
- Seasonings of choice

Directions:

1. Preheat your Smart Air Fryer Oven to 160°F.
2. Place the beef roast in a bowl and toss with olive oil and desired seasonings.
3. Put seasoned roast into the air fryer.
4. Select ROAST and set the temperature to 160°F, Time to 20 minutes.
5. Turn the roast when the Timer sounds and cook another 10 minutes.
6. Serve hot.

Nutrition: Calories 267 Fat 8 g Carbs 1 g Protein 21 g

Salt-and-Pepper Beef Roast

Preparation Time: 4 hours

Cooking Time: 30 minutes

Servings: 12-14

Ingredients:

- 4-6lbs boned beef cross rib roast
- 1/4 cup coarse salt
- 1/4 cup sugar
- 2 tbsp. coarse-ground pepper
- 1/2 cup horseradish

Directions:

1. Mix salt with sugar in a bowl. Pat the mixture on the beef, and marinate for 3-4 hours.
2. Mix 1.5 tsp. salt, pepper, and horseradish.
3. Put the beef on a rack in a 9"x13" pan and rub the horseradish mixture.
4. Roast in 1760C or 3500F in the Power XL Air Fryer Grill. Check if the internal temperature is 120-1250C.
5. Rest for 20 minutes, and then slice the meat thinly across the grain.

Nutrition: Calories: 267kcal, Carbs: 1.3g, Protein:

20g, Fat: 19g.

Prime Rib Roast

Preparation Time: 60 minutes

Cooking Time: 45 mins

Servings: 4-6

Ingredients:

- Prime Rib Roast
- Butter
- Salt and pepper

Directions:

1. Cut the fat parts from each side of the meat, and put it inside the Power XL Air Fryer Grill.
2. Cook at 2300C or 4500F for 15 minutes. Lower it to 1650C or 325 afterward.
3. Check if the internal temperature has reached 1100C or 2250F and serve.

Nutrition: Calories: 290kcal, Protein: 19.2g, Fat: 23.1g.

Beef Tenderloin

Preparation Time: 60 minutes

Cooking Time: 10 minutes

Servings: 6

Ingredients:

- 5 lbs. Beef Tenderloin
- Vegetable Oil
- Spices, salt, and pepper

Directions:

1. Preheat the Power XL Air Fryer Grill to 1800C or 3500F. Cut extra fat from it.
2. Gently rub tenderloin with vegetable oil and seasoning.
3. Cook it in the Power XL Air Fryer Grill for 20-30 mins.

Nutrition: Calories: 179kcal, Protein: 26g, Fat: 7.6g.

Perfect Rump Roast

Preparation Time: 2 hours

Cooking Time: 20 minutes

Servings: 5

Ingredients:

- 4lb rump roast
- 3 Garlic cloves
- 1 tbsp. each of salt, pepper
- 1 onion
- 1 cup water

Directions :

1. Preheat the Power XL Air Fryer Grill to 2600C or 5000F
2. Make 4-5 cuts on the roast, and fill with salt, pepper, and garlic.
3. Season some more before searing for 20 mins. Add water and minced onion.
4. Cook in the Power XL Air Fryer Grill at 1800C or 3500F for 1.5 hours.

Nutrition: Calories: 916.8kcal, Carbs: 4.4g, Protein: 94.6g, Fat: 55.2g.

Slow Roasted Beef Short Ribs

Preparation Time: 3 hours

Cooking Time: 10 minutes

Servings: 6

Ingredients:

- 5lbs beef short ribs
- 1/3 cup brown sugar
- 1 tsp. garlic powder
- 1 tsp. onion powder
- 1/4 tsp. marjoram
- 1/2 tsp. kosher salt
- 1/4 tsp. thyme
- 1 pinch cayenne pepper

Directions :

1. Pat the ribs dry.
2. Rub the Ingredients: on each rib, put them in a sealed plastic bag, and freeze overnight.
3. Preheat the Power XL Air Fryer Grill to 1500C or 3000F, and put ribs on a rack in a roasting pan.
4. Roast for around 3 hours.

Nutrition : Calories: 791kcal, Carbs: 19g, Protein: 79g, Fat: 42g.

Sirloin Roast Beef

Preparation Time: 90 minutes

Cooking Time: 15 minutes

Servings: 6

Ingredients:

- lbs. Sirloin of Beef
- 2 tbsp. vegetable oil
- 6 ounces red wine
- 14 ounces beef consommé

Directions:

1. Preheat the Power XL Air Fryer Grill to 2000C or 4000F.
2. Season the sirloin and cook it at medium heat in oil for 5 mins, turning regularly.
3. Roast it in the Power XL Air Fryer Grill for 15 mins to make it medium-rare. Flip it halfway.
4. Remove it when the internal temperature is 1450F, and cover with foil.
5. Make a gravy with the fat residue on the pan and some wine.

6. Add beef consommé to the sauce and simmer for 5 mins. Strain when completed and pour on the roast.

Nutrition: Calories: 179kcal, Protein: 22g, Fat: 9.4g.

Roasted Hamburgers

Preparation Time: 15 minutes

Cooking Time: 10 minutes

Servings: 6

Ingredients:

- 1-1/2 tsp. kosher salt
- 2 lbs. ground beef
- 1 tbsp. Worcestershire sauce
- 1/2 tsp. freshly ground black pepper
- 6 toasted hamburger buns
- Hamburger toppings

Directions:

1. Preheat the Power XL Air Fryer Grill to 2300C or 4500F, and line a rimmed baking sheet with aluminum foil with some salt to absorb drippings.
2. Season 1–2-inch lumps of meat by hand and split up meat into 6 parts to shape into 3"x1" disks
3. Place burgers an inch apart on a wire rack and roast for 10-16 mins at 1350C or 2500F for medium-rare meat.

Nutrition : Calories: 131.6kcal, Carbs: 8.7g, Protein:

13.1g, Fat: 4.1g.

Pan-Seared Roasted Strip Steak

Preparation Time: 20 minutes

Cooking Time: 10 minutes

Servings: 2

Ingredients:

- One 3-inch Strip Steak
- 1 tbsp. Butter
- Meat Tenderizer
- Coarsely Ground Black Pepper

Directions:

1. Cut and season the room-temperature meat.
2. Preheat the Power XL Air Fryer Grill to 2000C or 4000F.
3. Sear steak in butter over medium-high heat evenly for 2-3 mins after an hour of resting.
4. Cook in the Power XL Air Fryer Grill for 7 mins to achieve medium-rare.

Nutrition: Calories: 253.6kcal, Carbs: 0.2g, Protein: 21.1g, Fat: 18.1g,

London Broil Steak

Preparation Time: 50 minutes

Cooking Time: 20 minutes

Servings: 6

Ingredients:

2 lb. London broil top-round steak

Kosher salt

Freshly ground black pepper

1/4 cup extra-virgin olive oil

1/2 Lemon juice

2 tbsp. brown sugar

1 tbsp. Worcestershire sauce

4 cloves garlic, diced

1/4 cup Balsamic vinegar

Directions:

1. Marinate the steak in the refrigerator for at least 20 mins.
2. Preheat the Power XL Air Fryer Grill to 1900C or 3750F, and cook the steak for 6-8 mins on each side.

Nutrition: Calories: 173kcal, Protein: 26.1g, Fat: 7.7g.

Summer Sausage

Preparation Time: 40 minutes

Cooking Time:10 minutes

Serving: 6

Ingredients:

- 2-1/2 tsp of cracked black pepper
- 5 lb. of ground venison
- 3 tsp of tender quick salt
- 2-1/2 tsp of mustard seeds
- 1 tsp of liquid smoke
- 2-1/2 tsp of garlic salt
- 1 tsp of hickory salt

Directions:

1. In a bowl, mix ground venison, mustard seed, black pepper, and liquid smoke.
2. Add tender quick salt, garlic salt, and hickory salt.
3. Cut into 6 long rolls.
4. Place it on the Power XL Air Fryer Grill.
5. Set the Power XL Air Fryer Grill to broil function.
6. Cook for 4 hours at 1500F.
7. Serving Suggestions: serve with ketchup

8. Directions: & Cooking Tips: rinse venison well

Nutrition : Calories: 140kcal, Fat: 10g, Carb: 3g, Proteins: 13g

Meatball Venison

Preparation Time:10 minutes

Cooking Time: 30 minutes

Serving: 4

Ingredients:

- 1 tsp of salt
- 1 lb. of ground venison
- 1/2 tsp of nutmeg
- 1-1/2 can think of water
- 1 egg
- 1 cup of bread crumbs
- 1 can of mushroom soup
- 1/2 tsp of thyme
- 1 packet dried onion soup

Directions:

1. Mix salt, egg, meat, nutmeg, bread crumbs, and thyme in a bowl.
2. Shape into small balls
3. Place the meatball on the Power XL Air Fryer Grill pan.
4. Set the Power XL Air Fryer Grill to air fry function.
5. Cook for 30 minutes at 3500F.

6. Serve with mushroom soup

7. Serving Suggestions: Serve with dried onion soup

8. Directions: & Cooking Tips: rinse the meat well.

Nutrition: Calories: 57kcal, Fat: 2g, Carb: 2g, Proteins: 10g

Smoked Ham Sausage

Preparation time: 5 minutes

Cooking Time:5 minutes

Serving: 4

Ingredients:

- 1-1/2 tsp of sage
- Cayenne
- 1 tsp of thyme
- 3 lb. of venison
- 1 tsp of salt
- 1 lb. of smoked ham
- 1 tsp of ground pepper
- 1/2 lb. of bacon

Directions:

1. In a bowl, mix venison, thyme, sage, ground pepper, salt, and cayenne.
2. Cut the meats into pieces.
3. Mix all ingredients.
4. Shape platter out of it.
5. Place the platter on the Power XL Air Fryer Grill pan.
6. Set the Power XL Air Fryer Grill to broil function.

7. Cook for 15 minutes at 4000F

8. Serving Suggestions: serve with fries

9. Directions: & Cooking Tips: rinse meats well

Nutrition: Calories: 112kcal, Fat: 8g, Carb: 4g, Proteins: 10g

Venison Loaf

Preparation Time 1 hour

Cooking Time:10 minutes

Serving: 4

Ingredients:

- Chopped onion
- 1 lb. of sausage
- 1 cup of milk
- 2 eggs
- 8 ounces of barbecue sauce
- 2 cups of cracker crumbs
- Tomato sauce
- 1 lb. of ground venison

Directions:

1. Mix cracker crumbs, milk, ground venison, and barbecue sauce in a bowl.
2. Add sausage, eggs, and onion.
3. Place the mixture on the Power XL Air Fryer Grill pan.
4. Set the Power XL Air Fryer Grill to air fry function.
5. Bake for 1 hour at 3500F.

6. Serve immediately or allow cooling before serving
7. Serving Suggestions: Serve with tomato sauce
8. Directions: & Cooking Tips: mix the Ingredients: homogeneously.

Nutrition: Calories: kcal, fat: g, Carb: g, Proteins: g

Bologna

Preparation Time: 10 minutes

Cooking Time:45 minutes

Servings: 5

Ingredients:

- 1-1/2 tsp of liquid smoke
- 2 lb. of ground venison
- 1 cup of water
- 2 tbsp of tender-quick salt
- 1/2 tsp of garlic powder
- 4 tsp of onion powder

Directions:

1. Mix liquid smoke, garlic powder, water, and onion powder in a bowl.
2. Add tender-quick salt and ground venison.
3. Make rolls from the mixture.
4. Place the rolls on the Power XL Air Fryer Grill pan.
5. Set the Power XL Air Fryer Grill at broil function.
6. Cook for 45 minutes at 3000F.
7. Serving Suggestions: Serve with tomato sauce

8. Directions: & Cooking Tips: make the roll smooth

Nutrition: Calories: 249kcal, Fat: 21g, Carb: 1g, Proteins: 16g

Squirrel Dish

Preparation Time 40 minutes

Cooking Time:1 hour

Serving: 4

Ingredients:

- 1/2 cup of onion powder
- 1 can of tomatoes
- 1/2 dozen of potatoes
- 1 squirrel
- Vegetable oil
- Salt
- 1 cup of flour
- Pepper

Directions:

1. Cut the meats into cubes.
2. Add flour, salt, and pepper.
3. Add potatoes and onions.
4. Place the mixture on the Power XL Air Fryer Grill pan.
5. Set the Power XL Air Fryer Grill to air fry function
6. Cook for 1 hour 30 minutes at 3500F.
7. Serve immediately

8. Serving Suggestions: serve with tomato sauce

9. Directions: & Cooking Tips: rinse the squirrel meat well

Nutrition: Calories: 103kcal, Fat: 3g, Carb: 4g, Proteins: 19g

Swedish Meatballs

Preparation Time 40 minutes

Cooking Time:10minutes

Servings: 10

Ingredients:

- 1 pound ground beef
- 1 pound of ground pork
- 0.5 cup of panko breadcrumbs
- 0.5 onion, chopped
- 1 teaspoon of salt
- 0.5 teaspoon of ground black pepper
- 0.25 teaspoon nutmeg
- 1 teaspoon of garlic powder
- 1 teaspoon onion powder
- 1 egg
- 0.25 cup parsley, chopped
- 1.25 cups of cream, divided
- 2 tablespoons plus 2 teaspoons. Worcestershire sauce, divided
- 0.25 cup butter
- 0.25 cup of flour
- 3 cups of beef broth
- 1 sprig of fresh thyme

Directions:

1. Combine beef, pork, panko breadcrumbs, onion, salt, black pepper, nutmeg, garlic powder, onion powder, egg, parsley, ¼ cup heavy cream, and 2 teaspoons. Pour Worcestershire sauce into a bowl and use the mixture to form 30 meatballs.

2. Place the inner pot in the Power XL Fast Cooker.

3. Press the sauté button and then the program dial to select the beef set. Press the program selection again to confirm the default setting and start the cooking cycle (170 ° C for 20 minutes).

4. Put the butter in the inner pot and cook until the butter has melted.

5. Add flour and cook for 3 minutes.

6. Turn in the broth and simmer for not less than 10 to 11 minutes.

7. Click the Cancel button. Add the thyme, meatballs, and the rest of the Worcestershire cream and sauce.

8. Place the lid on the Power XL Quick Cooker and turn the lid counterclockwise. The lid is

locked and the pressure relief valve is closed.

9. Press the button, scroll to the meat setting, and press the program wheel. Press the Timer button, scroll to set the cooking Time to 4 minutes, and press the program wheel to start the cooking cycle.

10. When the Timer reaches 0, the Power XL Quick Pot will automatically switch to keep warm. Press the Cancel button. Let the Power XL Fast Cooker sit to naturally relieve the pressure. Turn the steam switch to open. Once the steam is released, the lid should be removed.

Nutrition: Calories: 42kcal, Fat: 0.5g, Carb: 10g, Proteins: 1g

Spaghetti and Meatballs

Preparation Time: 30 minutes

Cooking Time: 10 minutes

Servings: 8

Ingredients:

- 2 tablespoons of olive oil
- 1 small onion, chopped
- 6 cloves of garlic, chopped, divided
- 2 28-ounce cans of tomato paste
- 10 basil leaves
- 1 teaspoon of sea salt
- 1 spoon of sugar
- 1 teaspoon of ground black pepper, divided
- 0.5 cup chopped parsley, divided
- 2 pounds of ground beef
- 4 eggs
- 0.75 cup breadcrumbs
- 0.5 cup of milk
- 0.5 onion, chopped
- 1 teaspoon of salt
- 0.5 cup of grated parmesan cheese
- 1-pound cooked spaghetti

Directions:

1. Place the inner pot on the Power XL Fast Cooker.

2. Press the Sauté button, scroll to the Vegetable setting, and press the program selection. Press the Timer button, scroll to set the cooking Time to 20 minutes, and press the program wheel to start the cooking cycle.

3. Put olive oil, chopped onions, and 4 chopped garlic cloves in the inner pot and cook until translucent.

4. Add tomato puree, basil, sea salt, sugar, ½ teaspoon. Black pepper and ¼ cup parsley and cook for 10 minutes. Make the sauce. Press the Cancel button.

5. Mix the beef, eggs, breadcrumbs, milk, chopped onions, salt, parmesan, and the remaining garlic, black pepper, and parsley in a bowl and form meatballs from the mixture.

6. Place the meatballs in the hot sauce.

7. Place the lid on the Power XL Quick Cooker and turn the lid counter-clockwise. The lid

is locked and the pressure relief valve is closed.

8. Press the button, scroll to the meat setting, and press the program wheel. Press the Timer button, scroll to set the cooking Time to 20 minutes, and press the program wheel to start the cooking cycle.

9. When the Timer reaches, the Power XL Quick Pot will automatically switch to keeping warm. Press the Cancel button. Turn the steam release switch to open. Remove the lid once steam is released.

10. Remove the meatballs from the inner pot and serve over cooked spaghetti.

Nutrition: Calories: 57kcal, Fat: 2g, Carb: 2g, Proteins: 10g

BBQ Lamb

Preparation Time: 90 minutes

Cooking Time: 15 minutes

Servings: 8

Ingredients:

- 4 lbs. boneless leg of lamb, cut into 2-inch chunks
- 2-1/2 tbsps. herb salt
- 2 tbsps. olive oil

Directions:

1. Preheat the Power XL Air Fryer Grill by selecting air fryer mode
2. Adjust the temperature to 390°F, set Time to 5 minutes
3. Season the meat with salt and olive oil
4. Arrange on the Air fryer baking tray
5. Transfer to the Power XL Air Fryer Grill
6. Air fry for 15 minutes, flipping halfway through
7. Serve and enjoy
8. Serving Suggestions: serve with marinara sauce
9. Directions: & Cooking Tips: work in batches

Nutrition: Calories: 341kcal, Fat: 16g, Carb: 1g, Proteins: 26g

Lamb Meatballs

Preparation Time: 15minutes

Cooking Time: 15 minutes

Servings: 12

Ingredients:

- 1 lb. ground lamb
- 1/2 cup breadcrumbs
- 1 lemon, juiced and zested
- 1/4 cup milk
- 2 egg yolks
- 1 tsp ground cumin
- 1 tsp dried oregano
- 1/2 tsp salt
- 1 tsp ground coriander
- 1/2 tsp black pepper
- 3 garlic cloves, minced
- 1/4 cup fresh parsley, chopped
- 1/2 cup crumbled feta cheese

Directions:

1. Preheat the Power XL Air Fryer Grill by selecting Broil mode

2. Adjust the temperature to 390°F, set Time to 5 minutes
3. Combine all the ingredients in a bowl
4. Form into 12 balls
5. Arrange on the Air fryer baking tray
6. Transfer to the Power XL Air Fryer Grill
7. Cook for 12 minutes
8. Serve and enjoy
9. Serving Suggestions: Serve with tzatziki sauce
10. Directions: & Cooking Tips: rub olive oil on your hand when forming the meatballs

Nutrition: Calories: 129kcal, Fat: 6.4g, Carb: 4.9g, Proteins: 25g

Glazed Lamb Chops

Preparation Time: 30 minutes

Cooking Time: 15 minutes

Servings: 4

Ingredients:

- 4 (4-ounce) lamb loin chops
- 1 tbsp Dijon mustard
- 1 tsp honey
- 1/2 tbsp fresh lime juice
- 1/2 tsp olive oil
- Salt and ground black pepper, as required

Directions:

1. Preheat the Power XL Air Fryer Grill by selecting air fryer mode
2. Adjust the temperature to 3900 F, set Time to 5 minutes
3. Combine all the ingredients in a bowl
4. Add the pork chops and toss to coat
5. Arrange on the Air fryer baking tray
6. Transfer to the Power XL Air Fryer Grill
7. Air fry for 15 minutes, flipping halfway through
8. Serve and enjoy

9. Serving Suggestions: Serve while still hot

10. Directions: & Cooking Tips: leave to marinate for a few minutes

Nutrition: Calories: 224kcal, Fat: 4g, Carb: 2g, Proteins: 19g

Garlic Lamb Shank

Preparation Time: 15 minutes

Cooking Time: 24 minutes

Servings: 4

Ingredients:

- 17 oz. lamb shanks
- 2 tbsp garlic, peeled and coarsely chopped
- tsp kosher salt
- 1/2 cup chicken stock
- tbsp dried parsley
- 1 tsp dried rosemary
- 4 oz. chive stems, chopped
- 1 tsp butter
- 1 tsp nutmeg
- 1/2 tsp ground black pepper

Directions:

1. Make the cuts in the lamb shank and fill the cuts with the chopped garlic.
2. Sprinkle the lamb shank with the kosher salt, dried parsley, dried rosemary, nutmeg, and ground black pepper.
3. Stir the spices on the lamb shank gently.

4. Preheat the Power XL Air Fryer Grill by selecting air fry mode.
5. Adjust the temperature to 380°F, set Time to 5 minutes
6. put the butter, chives, and chicken stock in the air fryer baking tray.
7. Add the lamb shank and air fry the meat for 24 minutes.
8. Serve and enjoy
9. Serving Suggestions: Serve with the cooking liquid
10. Directions: & Cooking Tips: add spices to taste

Nutrition: Calories: 205kcal, Fat: 8.2g, Carb: 3g, Proteins: 28g

Indian Meatball with Lamb

Preparation Time: 10 minutes

Cooking Time: 14minutes

Servings: 8

Ingredients:

- 1 lb. ground lamb
- 1 garlic clove, minced
- 1 egg
- 1 tbsp butter
- 4 oz. chive stems, grated
- 1/4 tbsp turmeric
- 1/3 tsp cayenne pepper
- 1/4 tsp bay leaf
- 1 tsp ground coriander
- 1 tsp salt
- 1 tsp ground black pepper

Directions:

1. Combine all the ingredients together in a bowl
2. Preheat the Power XL air fryer by selecting the air fry mode
3. Adjust the temperature to 390°F and set Time to 5 minutes

4. Put the butter in the Air fryer baking tray and melt it.

5. Form the meatballs

6. Place them in the air fryer baking tray.

7. Transfer to the Power XL Air Fryer Grill

8. Cook the dish for 14 minutes.

9. Stir the meatballs twice during the cooking

10. Serving Suggestions: Serve with salad and sauce

11. Directions: & Cooking Tips: use an ice-cream scooper to form the balls

Nutrition : Calories: 300kcal, Fat: 13g, Carb: 19g, Proteins: 21g

Roasted Lamb

Preparation Time: 60 minutes

Cooking Time: 13 minutes

Servings: 4

Ingredients:

- 2-1/2 pounds lamb leg roast, slits carved
- tbsp olive oil
- garlic cloves, sliced into smaller slithers
- 1 tbsp dried rosemary
- Cracked Himalayan rock salt and cracked peppercorns, to taste

Directions:

1. Make the cuts in the lamb roast and insert them with garlic.
2. Sprinkle the lamb roast with kosher salt, rosemary, and ground black pepper.
3. Brush with oil.
4. Preheat the Power XL Air Fryer Grill by selecting air fry mode.
5. Adjust the temperature to 380°F, set Time to 5 minutes
6. Place the lamb roast on the Baking Pan
7. Transfer to the Power XL Air Fryer Grill.

8. Air fry for 1 hour 15 minutes

9. Serve and enjoy

10. Serving Suggestions: serve with mushroom sauce

11. Directions: & Cooking Tips: leave to marinate for some minutes

Nutrition: Calories: 246kcal, Fat: 7g, Carb: 9g, Proteins: 33g

Lamb Gyro

Preparation Time: 20 minutes

Cooking Time: 15 minutes

Servings: 4

Ingredients:

- 1 pound ground lamb
- 1/2 onion sliced
- 1/4 cup mint, minced
- 1/4 red onion, minced
- 1/8 tsp rosemary
- 1/2 tsp salt
- 1/2 tsp black pepper
- 3/4 cup hummus
- 4 slices pita bread
- 1/2 cucumber, peeled and sliced into thin rounds
- 1 cup romaine lettuce, shredded
- 1 Roma tomato, diced
- 1/4 cup parsley, minced
- 2 cloves garlic, minced
- 12 mint leaves, minced

Directions:

1. Preheat the Power XL Air Fryer Grill by selecting broil mode
2. Adjust the temperature to 3700F, set Time to 5 minutes
3. Mix lamb with onions, mint, parsley, garlic, salt, rosemary, and pepper
4. Form into patties
5. Arrange in a lined Air fryer baking tray
6. Transfer to the Power XL Air Fryer Grill
7. Air fry for 20 minutes, flipping halfway through
8. Assemble the gyro with the remaining Ingredients:
9. Serve and enjoy
10. Serving Suggestions: serve drizzled with tzatziki sauce
11. Directions: & Cooking Tips: mix until well incorporated

Nutrition: Calories: 309kcal, Fat: 14.6g, Carb: 29g, Proteins: 19g

Lemon Lamb Rack

Preparation Time: 30 minutes

Cooking Time: 10 minutes

Servings: 4

Ingredients:

- 1/4 cup olive oil
- 3 tbsp garlic, minced
- 1/3 cup dry white wine
- 1 tbsp lemon zest, grated
- 2 tbsps. lemon juice
- 1-1/2 tsp dried oregano, crushed
- 1 tsp thyme leaves, minced
- Salt and black pepper
- 4 lamb rack
- 1 lemon, sliced

Directions:

1. Whisk everything in a baking pan to coat the chicken breasts well.
2. Place the lemon slices on top of the chicken breasts.
3. Spread the mustard mixture over the toasted bread slices.

4. Press "Power Button" of Air Fry Oven and turn the dial to select the "Bake" mode.
5. Press the Time button and again turn the dial to set the cooking Time to 30 minutes.
6. Now push the Temp button and rotate the dial to set the temperature at 370 degrees F.
7. Once preheated, place the baking pan inside and close its lid.
8. Serve warm.
9. Directions:
10. Preheat the Power XL Air Fryer Grill by selecting air fryer mode
11. Adjust the temperature to 3700F, set Time to 5 minutes
12. Whisk all the ingredients together in a bowl
13. Pour into air fryer baking tray
14. Add the lamb rack
15. Top with lemon
16. Transfer to the Power XL Air Fryer Grill
17. Air fry for 30 minutes, flipping halfway through
18. Serve and enjoy

19. Serving Suggestions: Serve with the juice

20. Directions: & Cooking Tips: Leave to marinate for a few minutes

Nutrition: Calories: 288kcal, Fat: 7g, Carb: 5g, Proteins: 16g

Juicy & Savory Lamb Chops

Preparation Time:10 minutes

Cooking Time: 10 minutes

Servings:1

Ingredients:

- 1/3 lb. lamb chop
- 1 tbsp mixed fresh herbs, chopped
- 1/2 tbsp olive oil
- 1/2 tbsp Dijon mustard
- Pepper
- Salt

Directions:

1. Season lamb chop with pepper and salt.
2. In a small bowl, mix together oil, mustard, and mixed herbs.
3. Brush lamb chop from both the sides with oil mixture.
4. Place lamb chop into the air fryer basket and cook at 375 F for 10 minutes. Turn halfway through.

Nutrition: Calories 350 Fat 18.5 g Carbohydrates 1.2 g Sugar 0.1 g Protein 43 g Cholesterol 136 mg

Lamb Patties

Preparation Time: 10 minutes

Cooking Time: 30 minutes

Servings: 4

Ingredients:

- 1 lb. ground lamb meat
- 1 egg, lightly beaten
- 1/2 tbsp garlic, minced
- 1 spring onion, chopped
- 1/4 cup almond flour
- 1 tbsp basil, chopped
- 1 tbsp cilantro, chopped
- Pepper
- Salt

Directions:

1. Spray air fryer basket with cooking spray.
2. Add all Ingredients into the bowl and mix until well combined.
3. Make small patties from meat mixture and place into the air fryer basket and cook at 390 F for 30 minutes. Turn patties halfway through.
4. Serve and enjoy.

Nutrition: Calories 260 Fat 17 g Carbohydrates 1.1 g Sugar 0.2 g Protein 23 g Cholesterol 121 mg

Rosemary Lamb Chops

Preparation Time:10 minutes

Cooking Time: 12 minutes

Servings:2

Ingredients:

- 4 lamb chops
- 2 tsp ginger garlic paste
- 2 tsp olive oil
- 1 tsp rosemary, chopped
- Pepper
- Salt

Directions:

1. Add lamb chops, ginger garlic paste, oil, rosemary, pepper, and salt into the zip-lock bag.
2. Seal bag shake well and place it in the refrigerator for 1 hour.
3. Add marinated lamb chops into the air fryer basket and cook at 360 F for 12 minutes. Turn halfway through.
4. Serve and enjoy.

Nutrition: Calories 461 Fat 22.3 g Carbohydrates 3.4 g Sugar 0 g Protein 64.2 g Cholesterol 203 mg

Dijon Garlic Lamb Chops

Preparation Time:10 minutes

Cooking Time: 17 minutes

Servings:4

Ingredients:

- 8 lamb chops
- 1 tsp cayenne pepper
- 1 tsp cumin powder
- 1 tsp garlic, minced
- 1 tsp soy sauce
- 2 tsp olive oil
- 2 tsp Dijon mustard
- 1/4 tsp salt

Directions:

1. Add lamb chops and remaining Ingredients into the zip-lock bag. Seal bag shake well and place it in the refrigerator for 30 minutes.
2. Place marinated lamb chops into the air fryer basket and cook at 350 F for 17 minutes. Turn lamb chops halfway through.
3. Serve and enjoy.

Nutrition: Calories 445 Fat 19.1 g Carbohydrates 0.9

g Sugar 0.1 g Protein 63.6 g Cholesterol 203 mg

www.ingramcontent.com/pod-product-compliance
Lightning Source LLC
Chambersburg PA
CBHW050758030426
42336CB00012B/1868